Cough No More

Natural Cough Remedies for Adults to Soothe and Heal

Isabella White

Copyright © 2023 by Isabella White.

All rights reserved. No part of this publication may be reproduced, distributed, or transmitted in any form or by any means, including photocopying, recording, or other electronic or mechanical methods, without the prior written permission of the publisher, except in the case of brief quotations embodied in critical reviews and certain other noncommercial uses permitted by copyright law.

Disclaimer: The information contained in this book is based on the research, opinions, and experiences of the author. It is not intended to replace professional medical advice or treatment. The reader should regularly consult a physician for any health issues and always seek the advice of a physician before modifying diet, supplement, or exercise regimens.

The author and publisher shall have neither liability nor responsibility to any person or entity concerning any loss or damage related to the information contained in this book. The information provided is general in nature and may not apply to every individual. Any reliance on the information contained herein is solely at the reader's own risk.

Contents

Chapter 5

Introduction

Coughing is one of the most common reasons adults seek medical care. Whether you have an annoying dry cough or a phlegm-producing cough that won't quit, coughs can disrupt your life and rob you of much-needed rest.

When that dreaded cough strikes, you want fast-acting, safe relief. But with all the over-the-counter medications out there with long lists of side effects, where do you turn? A growing body of research shows that natural remedies can be just as effective for cough relief, minus the risks and complications of prescription medications.

In *Cough No More: Natural Cough Remedies for Adults to Soothe and Heal,* you'll learn what works when it comes to naturally calming coughs. You'll understand the different types of coughs, their underlying causes, and when to seek professional treatment. You'll discover time-tested natural ingredients that can help tame even the most stubborn coughs. From lifestyle adjustments to herbal remedies to soothing DIY concoctions, this book offers natural solutions to put an end to your cough woes.

Say goodbye to sleepless nights and irritating coughing fits! With the holistic, evidence-based treatments in this book, you'll be armed with the knowledge you need to stop coughs in their tracks—the natural way. Breathe easy and reclaim your comfort, health, and peace of mind.

Chapter 1

Understanding Cough and Its Causes

What is a Cough?

A cough is a reflex action that helps to clear the airways of irritants, mucus, and foreign substances. A variety of respiratory conditions can cause shortness of breath, which can be influenced by several factors. Coughing is the body's way of protecting the lungs and airways from potential harm.

When you cough, your body forcefully expels air from your lungs, creating a sudden burst of sound. This action helps to remove any irritants or excess mucus that may be present in the respiratory system. Coughing can be voluntary or involuntary, and it can occur in short bursts or persist for longer periods.

Coughs can vary in intensity, duration, and sound. They can be dry or productive, meaning they produce phlegm or mucus. While productive coughs typically result from excessive mucus production as a result of an infection or other respiratory condition, dry coughs are frequently brought on by irritation or inflammation in the throat or airways.

Coughs can be acute or chronic. A viral infection, like the common cold or the flu, is typically what causes acute coughs, which can last anywhere from a few days to a few weeks. Chronic coughs, on the other hand, persist for more than eight weeks and can be a sign of an underlying medical condition, such as asthma, allergies, or gastroesophageal reflux disease (GERD).

Coughs, in addition to being a symptom of respiratory conditions, can also be triggered by environmental factors such as exposure to smoke, dust, or strong odors. Other common causes of coughing in adults include postnasal drip, sinusitis, allergies, and certain medications.

It's important to note that coughing itself is not a disease but rather a symptom of an underlying condition. Therefore, it's crucial to identify and address the root cause of the cough to effectively treat it.

Coughing is sometimes accompanied by other symptoms such as chest congestion, wheezing, shortness of breath, or fever. These additional symptoms can provide valuable clues about the underlying cause of the cough and help guide appropriate treatment.

While most coughs are not serious and resolve on their own with time, there are instances when medical attention should be sought. If you experience any of the following, it is advisable to consult a healthcare professional:

- Coughing up blood or bloody mucus
- Chest pain or tightness
- Difficulty breathing or shortness of breath
- High fever
- Persistent cough lasting more than three weeks
- Cough accompanied by unexplained weight loss
- Cough that worsens or does not improve with time

These symptoms may indicate a more serious underlying condition that requires medical evaluation and treatment.

In the next section, we will explore the common causes of cough in adults, helping you gain a better understanding of what might be triggering your cough and how to address it effectively.

Common Causes of Cough in Adults

Coughing is a common symptom caused by a variety of factors. Understanding the underlying causes of your cough can help you find the most effective remedies to soothe and heal it. In this section, we will explore some of the common causes of cough in adults.

1. Upper Respiratory Infections

One of the most common causes of cough in adults is an upper respiratory infection, such as the common cold or flu. These infections can irritate the throat and airways, leading to a persistent cough. The cough may start off dry and later become productive, producing mucus or phlegm. Other symptoms that may accompany an upper respiratory infection include nasal congestion, a sore throat, and fatigue.

2. Allergies

Allergies can also trigger coughing in adults. When you are exposed to allergens such as pollen, dust mites, or pet dander, your immune system reacts by releasing histamines. These histamines can cause inflammation in the airways, leading to coughing and other allergy symptoms. Allergic coughs are often accompanied by other symptoms like sneezing, itchy eyes, and a runny nose.

3. Asthma

Asthma is a chronic condition that affects the airways and can cause coughing. When a person with asthma is exposed to triggers such as allergens, exercise, or cold air, their airways become inflamed and narrow, making it difficult to breathe. Coughing is a common symptom of asthma and can be triggered by exercise or exposure to irritants. Other symptoms of asthma may include wheezing, shortness of breath, and chest tightness.

4. Gastroesophageal reflux disease (GERD)

GERD is a condition in which stomach acid flows back into the esophagus, causing irritation and inflammation. This can lead to a chronic cough, known as a reflux cough. The cough is often worse at night or after eating and may be accompanied by heartburn or a sour taste in the mouth. Treating GERD can help alleviate the cough symptoms.

5. Postnasal drip

Postnasal drip occurs when excess mucus from the nose drips down the back of the throat. This can irritate the throat and trigger a cough. Postnasal drip can be caused by allergies, sinus infections, or even weather changes. Along with coughing, you may experience a tickling sensation in the throat, a constant need to clear your throat, and a runny or stuffy nose.

6. Smoking

Smoking is a major cause of cough in adults. The chemicals in tobacco smoke can irritate the airways and lead to chronic bronchitis, a condition characterized by a persistent cough with mucus production. Quitting smoking is essential for improving respiratory health and reducing coughing episodes.

7. Environmental irritants

Exposure to environmental irritants such as air pollution, dust, or strong odors can also cause coughing in adults. These irritants can irritate the airways and trigger a cough reflex. If you work in an environment with high levels of pollutants or chemicals, it is important to take precautions to minimize exposure and protect your respiratory health.

8. Medications

Certain medications, such as ACE inhibitors used to treat high blood pressure, can cause a persistent cough as a side effect. If you suspect that your cough may be caused by a medication you are taking, it is important to consult with your healthcare provider to explore alternative options.

9. Chronic obstructive pulmonary disease (COPD)

COPD is a progressive lung disease that includes chronic bronchitis and emphysema. Coughing is a common symptom of COPD and is often accompanied by shortness of breath, wheezing, and chest tightness. If you have a history of smoking or exposure to lung irritants, it is important to get evaluated for COPD if you experience a persistent cough.

10. Other causes

In some cases, a cough may be caused by less common factors such as lung infections, lung cancer, or certain autoimmune conditions. If your cough is persistent, severe, or accompanied by other concerning symptoms, it is important to seek medical attention for a proper evaluation and diagnosis.

Understanding the common causes of cough in adults can help you identify the root cause of your cough and choose the most appropriate remedies for relief. In the next section, we will discuss when it is necessary to seek medical attention for a cough.

When to Seek Medical Attention for a Cough

While most coughs are harmless and will go away on their own, there are certain situations where seeking medical attention for a cough is necessary. It's important to be aware of the warning signs that indicate a more serious underlying condition. This section will guide you on when it's appropriate to consult a healthcare professional for your cough.

Persistent or Worsening Cough

If your cough persists for more than three weeks or is getting worse instead of improving, it's time to seek medical attention. A persistent cough could be a sign of an underlying health issue that needs to be addressed. It could be caused by conditions such as asthma, chronic bronchitis, or even lung cancer. A healthcare professional will be able to evaluate your symptoms, perform necessary tests, and provide appropriate treatment.

Cough Accompanied by Severe Symptoms

If your cough is accompanied by severe symptoms, it's important to seek medical attention promptly. Severe symptoms may include:

- **High fever:** A persistent cough with a high fever could be a sign of a respiratory infection such as pneumonia. Prompt medical attention is necessary to prevent complications.

- **Shortness of breath:** If your cough is causing difficulty breathing or you feel like you can't catch your breath, it could be a sign of a more serious respiratory condition. Seek immediate medical attention in such cases.

- **Chest pain:** If your cough is accompanied by chest pain, it could be a sign of a more serious condition such as pneumonia, bronchitis, or even a heart problem. It's important to get evaluated by a healthcare professional to determine the cause of the chest pain.

- **Coughing up blood:** If you are coughing up blood or noticing blood in your phlegm, it's crucial to seek immediate medical attention. This could be a sign of a serious underlying condition that needs to be addressed urgently.

Cough Lasting More than Eight Weeks

If your cough persists for more than eight weeks, it is considered a chronic cough. Chronic coughs can be caused by various factors, such as postnasal drip, acid reflux, or even certain medications. However, it's important to consult a healthcare professional to determine the underlying cause and receive appropriate treatment. They may recommend further tests or refer you to a specialist if necessary.

Cough in Individuals with Pre-existing Health Conditions

If you have a pre-existing health condition such as asthma, chronic obstructive pulmonary disease (COPD), or a weakened immune system, it's important to seek medical attention for your cough. These conditions can make you more susceptible to respiratory infections and complications. A healthcare professional will be able to assess your symptoms, provide appropriate treatment, and help manage your condition effectively.

Cough in Children or Older Adults

Coughs in children and older adults can be more concerning due to their weaker immune systems and increased vulnerability to respiratory infections. If a child under the age of six months has a cough, it's important to seek medical attention as their immune systems are still developing. Similarly, if an older adult has a persistent or worsening cough, it's advisable to consult a healthcare professional to rule out any serious underlying conditions.

Cough with Other Concerning Symptoms

If your cough is accompanied by other concerning symptoms such as unexplained weight loss, night sweats, fatigue, or a persistent hoarse voice, it's important to seek medical attention. These symptoms could be indicative of a more serious underlying condition that requires evaluation and treatment.

Remember, it's always better to err on the side of caution when it comes to your health. If you are unsure about the severity of your cough or if it's causing significant distress, it's best to consult a healthcare professional. They will be able to assess your symptoms, provide an accurate diagnosis, and recommend appropriate treatment options to help you find relief from your cough.

Preventing Cough and Maintaining Respiratory Health

Preventing cough and maintaining respiratory health are essential for overall well-being. While it's not always possible to completely avoid coughs, there are steps you can take to reduce the risk and keep your respiratory system in good shape. In this section, we will explore some preventive measures and lifestyle habits that can help you maintain a healthy respiratory system.

1. Practice good hygiene.

One of the most effective ways to prevent coughs and respiratory infections is by practicing good hygiene. This includes washing your hands frequently with soap and water for at least 20 seconds, especially before eating or touching your face. Avoid close contact with people who have a cough or cold, and cover your mouth and nose with a tissue or your elbow when coughing or sneezing to prevent the spread of germs.

2. Maintain a clean and healthy environment.

Keeping your living and working spaces clean and free from allergens can significantly reduce the risk of coughs and respiratory issues. Regularly dust and vacuum your home, especially areas where dust tends to accumulate, such as carpets, curtains, and upholstery. Use a damp cloth when dusting to prevent the particles from becoming airborne. Additionally, ensure proper ventilation in your home to improve air quality and reduce the concentration of pollutants.

3. Avoid smoking and secondhand smoke.

Smoking is one of the leading causes of respiratory problems, including chronic cough. If you smoke, the best thing you can do for your respiratory health is to quit. Smoking weakens your immune system and damages your lungs, increasing your risk of developing respiratory infections. Additionally, exposure to secondhand smoke can also irritate the airways and trigger coughing. Avoiding both active and passive smoking is crucial for maintaining a healthy respiratory system.

4. Stay hydrated.

Proper hydration is essential for maintaining respiratory health. Drinking an adequate amount of water helps keep the mucus membranes in your respiratory tract moist, which can help prevent coughs and soothe irritated airways. Aim to drink at least 8 glasses of water per day, and increase your fluid intake if you have a cough or respiratory infection. Avoid excessive consumption of caffeinated and sugary beverages, as they can dehydrate the body.

5. Eat a balanced diet.

A healthy diet plays a vital role in supporting respiratory health. Include a variety of fruits, vegetables, whole grains, and lean proteins in your meals to provide your body with essential nutrients and antioxidants. These nutrients help strengthen the immune system and reduce the risk of respiratory infections. Incorporate foods rich in vitamin C, such as citrus fruits, berries, and leafy greens, as they have been shown to support respiratory health. Avoid excessive consumption of processed foods, sugary snacks, and drinks, as they can weaken the immune system and contribute to inflammation.

6. Exercise regularly.

Regular exercise not only benefits your cardiovascular system but also helps maintain respiratory health. Engaging in physical activity improves lung function, increases lung capacity, and enhances overall respiratory efficiency. On most days of the week, try to get in at least 30 minutes of moderate-intensity exercise, such as brisk walking, cycling, or swimming. If you have a chronic cough or respiratory condition, consult your healthcare professional before starting any exercise program.

7. Manage stress.

Stress can hurt your respiratory health and increase the likelihood of developing a cough. When you are stressed, your body releases stress hormones, which can weaken your immune system and make you more susceptible to respiratory infections. To reduce stress, practice stress-reduction techniques such as deep breathing exercises, meditation, yoga, or engaging in activities that you enjoy. Getting enough rest and sleep is also crucial for managing stress and maintaining a healthy respiratory system.

8. Avoid allergens and irritants.

If you have allergies, it's important to identify and avoid triggers that can cause coughing and respiratory symptoms.

Common allergens include pollen, dust mites, pet dander, and mold. Take steps to minimize your exposure to these allergens by keeping your home clean, using allergen-proof bedding covers, and avoiding outdoor activities during peak pollen seasons. If necessary, consult an allergist for further evaluation and guidance on managing your allergies.

9. Stay up-to-date with vaccinations.

Vaccinations can help prevent certain respiratory infections, such as influenza and pneumonia. Make sure you are up to date with your vaccinations, especially if you are at a higher risk of complications from respiratory infections, such as older adults or individuals with chronic health conditions. Consult your healthcare professional to determine which vaccinations are recommended for you based on your age, health status, and other factors.

By following these preventive measures and incorporating healthy habits into your lifestyle, you can reduce the risk of coughs and maintain optimal respiratory health. However, if you do develop a cough or respiratory symptoms that persist or worsen, it's important to seek medical attention to rule out any underlying conditions and receive appropriate treatment.

Chapter 2

Natural Remedies for Cough Relief

Herbal Remedies for Soothing a Cough

When it comes to soothing a cough, nature has provided us with a treasure trove of herbal remedies that can help alleviate symptoms and promote healing. These natural remedies have been used for centuries and are known for their effectiveness in soothing irritated throats, reducing coughing spasms, and supporting respiratory health. In this section, we will explore some of the most popular herbal remedies for cough relief.

1. Marshmallow Root

Marshmallow root, also known as Althaea officinalis, is a herb that has been used for centuries to soothe coughs and sore throats. It contains mucilage, a gel-like substance that coats the throat and provides relief from irritation. Marshmallow root can be consumed as a tea or taken in supplement form. To make marshmallow root tea, steep 1-2 teaspoons of dried marshmallow root in a cup of hot water for 10–15 minutes. Drink this tea 2-3 times a day to soothe your cough and ease throat discomfort.

2. Licorice Root

Licorice root, or Glycyrrhiza glabra, is another herbal remedy that has been used for centuries to soothe coughs and respiratory ailments. It contains compounds that have expectorant properties, helping to loosen mucus and relieve congestion. Licorice root can be consumed as a tea or taken in supplement form. To make licorice root tea, steep 1-2 teaspoons of dried licorice root in a cup of hot water for 10–15 minutes. Drink this tea 2-3 times a day to help soothe your cough and promote respiratory health.

3. Thyme

Thyme, or Thymus vulgaris, is a fragrant herb that is not only delicious in cooking but also has medicinal properties. It contains compounds that have antitussive and expectorant effects, making it an excellent herbal remedy for cough relief. Thyme can be consumed as tea or used in steam inhalation. To make thyme tea, steep 1-2 teaspoons of dried thyme leaves in a cup of hot water for 10–15 minutes. Drink this tea 2-3 times a day to help soothe your cough and clear congestion. For steam inhalation, add a few drops of thyme essential oil to a bowl of hot water, cover your head with a towel, and inhale the steam for 10-15 minutes.

4. Eucalyptus

Eucalyptus, or Eucalyptus globulus, is a powerful herbal remedy for cough relief due to its expectorant and decongestant properties. It contains a compound called cineole, which helps to loosen mucus and relieve coughing. Eucalyptus can be used for steam inhalation or applied topically as a chest rub. For steam inhalation, add a few drops of eucalyptus essential oil to a bowl of hot water, cover your head with a towel, and inhale the steam for 10-15 minutes. For a chest rub, dilute eucalyptus essential oil with carrier oil, such as coconut oil, and massage it onto your chest and throat.

5. Ginger

Ginger, or Zingiber officinale, is a versatile herb that has been used for centuries in traditional medicine for its numerous health benefits. It has anti-inflammatory and antimicrobial properties, making it an excellent herbal remedy for soothing a cough. Ginger can be consumed as a tea or added to foods and beverages. To make ginger tea, steep 1-2 teaspoons of grated fresh ginger in a cup of hot water for 10–15 minutes. Drink this tea 2-3 times a day to help soothe your cough and reduce inflammation in your respiratory system.

6. Slippery Elm Bark

Slippery elm bark, or Ulmus rubra, is a herb that has been used for centuries by Native Americans to soothe coughs and sore throats. It contains mucilage, which forms a protective coating on the throat and helps to reduce irritation and coughing. Slippery elm bark can be consumed as a tea or taken in supplement form. To make slippery elm bark tea, mix 1-2 teaspoons of powdered slippery elm bark with hot water to make a thick paste. Gradually add more hot water to the paste, stirring constantly, until you reach the desired consistency. Drink this tea 2-3 times a day to help soothe your cough and relieve throat discomfort.

7. Mullein

Mullein, or Verbascum thapsus, is a herb that has been used for centuries to soothe coughs and respiratory ailments. It has expectorant and anti-inflammatory properties, making it an effective herbal remedy for cough relief. Mullein can be consumed as a tea or used in steam inhalation. To make mullein tea, steep 1-2 teaspoons of dried mullein leaves in a cup of hot water for 10–15 minutes. Drink this tea 2-3 times a day to help soothe your cough and reduce inflammation in your respiratory system. For steam inhalation, add a few drops of mullein essential oil to a bowl of hot water, cover your head with a towel, and inhale the steam for 10-15 minutes.

These herbal remedies can be a valuable addition to your cough relief arsenal. However, it's important to note that everyone's body is different, and what works for one person may not work for another. If you have any underlying health conditions or are taking medication, it's always a good idea to consult with a healthcare professional before incorporating herbal remedies into your cough relief routine.

Essential Oils for Cough Relief

Essential oils have been used for centuries for their therapeutic properties and are known for their ability to provide relief from various ailments, including coughs. These oils are derived from plants and contain concentrated compounds that can help soothe and heal the respiratory system. In this section, we will explore some of the most effective essential oils for cough relief and how to use them.

1. Eucalyptus oil

Eucalyptus oil is one of the most popular essential oils for respiratory health. It contains a compound called cineole, which has been shown to have anti-inflammatory and expectorant properties. These properties make eucalyptus oil effective in relieving coughs and congestion.

To use eucalyptus oil for cough relief, add a few drops to a diffuser or humidifier and inhale the steam. Alternately, you could combine some eucalyptus oil with a carrier oil, like coconut oil, and massage your chest and throat with the mixture. This can help open up the airways and reduce coughing.

2. Peppermint oil

Peppermint oil is another essential oil that is commonly used for cough relief. It contains menthol, which has a cooling effect and can help to soothe irritated airways. Peppermint oil also has antimicrobial properties, which can aid in the fight against respiratory infections that may be causing the cough.

To use peppermint oil for cough relief, you can add a few drops to a bowl of hot water and inhale the steam. This can help to clear congestion and reduce coughing. You can also mix a few drops of peppermint oil with a carrier oil and apply it to your chest and throat for added relief.

3. Tea tree oil

Tea tree oil is well-known for its antimicrobial properties and is often used to treat respiratory infections. It can help kill off bacteria and viruses that may be causing the cough. Tea tree oil also has expectorant properties, which can help to loosen mucus and phlegm, making it easier to cough up.

To use tea tree oil for cough relief, you can add a few drops to a diffuser or humidifier and inhale the steam. You can also mix a few drops with carrier oil and apply it to your chest and throat. However, it's important to note that tea tree oil should not be ingested, as it can be toxic if swallowed.

4. Lavender oil

Lavender oil is known for its calming and soothing properties, making it a great choice for relieving coughs that are accompanied by stress or anxiety. It can help to relax the muscles in the respiratory system and reduce coughing.

To use lavender oil for cough relief, you can add a few drops to a diffuser or inhale it directly from the bottle. You can also mix a few drops with carrier oil and apply it to your chest and throat for added relaxation.

5. Lemon oil

Lemon oil is a powerful immune booster and can help fight off respiratory infections that may be causing the cough. It also has expectorant properties, which can help to loosen mucus and phlegm.

To use lemon oil for cough relief, you can add a few drops to a diffuser or inhale it directly from the bottle. You can also mix a few drops with carrier oil and apply it to your chest and throat. Additionally, you can add a few drops of lemon oil to a cup of warm water and gargle with it to soothe a sore throat.

6. Other essential oils for cough relief

In addition to the essential oils mentioned above, several others can provide relief from coughs. These include:

- **Frankincense oil:** Known for its anti-inflammatory properties, frankincense oil can help reduce inflammation in the respiratory system and alleviate coughing.
- **Thyme oil:** Thyme oil has antimicrobial properties and can help fight off respiratory infections. It also has expectorant properties, making it effective in relieving coughs.
- **Rosemary oil:** Rosemary oil has antispasmodic properties, which can help to relax the muscles in the respiratory system and reduce coughing.
- **Oregano oil:** Oregano oil is a potent antimicrobial and can help to kill off bacteria and viruses that may be causing the cough.

When using essential oils for cough relief, it's important to dilute them with carrier oil before applying them to the skin. This helps to prevent skin irritation. It's also a good idea to do a patch test before using any essential oil to ensure that you are not allergic to it.

Home Remedies Using Common Kitchen Ingredients

When it comes to finding relief from a cough, you don't always have to look further than your kitchen. Many common ingredients found in your pantry can be used as effective home remedies to soothe and heal your cough. These remedies are not only natural but also easily accessible and affordable. In this section, we will explore some of these kitchen ingredients and how they can help alleviate your cough symptoms.

1. Honey

Honey has been used for centuries as a natural cough and sore throat remedy. Its soothing properties can help relieve throat irritation and inflammation, resulting in less coughing. Honey also contains antimicrobial properties, which can aid in the fight against infections that may be causing your cough.

To use honey as a cough remedy, you can mix it with warm water or herbal tea. Add a tablespoon of honey to a cup of warm water or tea and stir until the honey is dissolved. Sip on this mixture throughout the day to soothe your cough and provide relief.

2. Ginger

Ginger is another powerful ingredient that can help alleviate cough symptoms. It has anti-inflammatory properties that can help to reduce throat and airway irritation, which can help to suppress coughing. Additionally, ginger has antimicrobial properties that can protect against respiratory infections.

To use ginger as a cough remedy, you can make ginger tea. Grate some fresh ginger, then let it steep in hot water for about ten minutes. Strain the tea and add a teaspoon of honey for added soothing benefits. Drink this ginger tea a few times a day to help relieve your cough.

3. Garlic

Garlic is well-known for its immune-boosting properties, but it can also be beneficial in relieving cough symptoms. Garlic contains compounds that have antimicrobial and expectorant properties, which can help fight off infections and loosen mucus in the airways.

To use garlic as a cough remedy, you can make garlic-infused honey. Crush a few cloves of garlic and mix them with a tablespoon of honey. Let the mixture sit for a few hours to allow the garlic to infuse into the honey. Take a teaspoon of this mixture a few times a day to help soothe your cough.

4. Turmeric

Turmeric is a spice commonly used in cooking, but it also has medicinal properties that can help alleviate cough symptoms. It contains curcumin, a compound with anti-inflammatory and antioxidant properties. These properties can help reduce inflammation in the airways and soothe coughing.

To use turmeric as a cough remedy, you can make a turmeric milk drink. Heat a cup of milk and add a teaspoon of turmeric powder. Stir well and add a pinch of black pepper to enhance the absorption of curcumin. Drink this turmeric milk before bedtime to help relieve your cough and promote restful sleep.

5. Lemon

Lemon is a citrus fruit that is rich in vitamin C and antioxidants. It can help boost your immune system and fight off infections that may be causing your cough. Lemon also has a soothing effect on the throat and can help reduce coughing.

To use lemon as a cough remedy, you can make a lemon and honey drink. Squeeze the juice of half a lemon into a cup of warm water and add a tablespoon of honey. Stir well, and drink this mixture a few times a day to help soothe your cough.

6. Saltwater gargle

A saltwater gargle is a simple yet effective remedy for soothing a cough and relieving throat irritation. Saltwater can help reduce inflammation and kill bacteria in the throat, providing relief from coughing.

To make a saltwater gargle, dissolve half a teaspoon of salt in a cup of warm water. Gargle with this mixture for about 30 seconds, then spit it out. Repeat this several times a day to help alleviate your cough.

7. Steam inhalation

Steam inhalation can help relieve congestion and soothe a cough by moisturizing the airways. It can also help loosen mucus, making it easier to expel.

To do steam inhalation, fill a bowl with hot water and add a few drops of essential oils, such as eucalyptus or peppermint. Lean over the bowl, cover your head with a towel to trap the steam, and inhale deeply for about 10 minutes. Be cautious to avoid burning yourself with the hot water. Repeat this a few times a day to help relieve your cough.

These home remedies using common kitchen ingredients can provide effective relief for your cough symptoms. However, it's important to note that if your cough persists for more than a few weeks or is accompanied by other severe symptoms, it's advisable to seek medical attention.

Alternative Therapies for Cough Relief

While herbal remedies, essential oils, and home remedies can be effective in soothing and relieving cough symptoms, there are also alternative therapies that can provide additional relief. These therapies focus on promoting overall wellness and addressing the underlying causes of cough. In this section, we will explore some alternative therapies that can complement traditional cough remedies.

Acupuncture

Acupuncture is an ancient Chinese practice that involves inserting thin needles into specific points on the body. It is believed to stimulate the body's natural healing processes and restore balance. Acupuncture has been used for centuries to treat various ailments, including cough.

When it comes to cough relief, acupuncture can help by targeting the underlying imbalances in the body that may be contributing to the cough. By stimulating specific acupuncture points, it can help to strengthen the immune system, reduce inflammation, and promote respiratory health. Acupuncture may also help to alleviate cough-related symptoms such as chest congestion and throat irritation.

If you are considering acupuncture for cough relief, it is important to consult with a qualified and experienced acupuncturist. They will be able to assess your condition and develop a personalized treatment plan tailored to your specific needs.

Breathing Exercises

Breathing exercises can be a valuable tool for managing and reducing cough symptoms. These exercises focus on improving lung function, promoting relaxation, and reducing stress, all of which can contribute to cough relief.

One effective breathing exercise for cough relief is diaphragmatic breathing. This technique involves deep breathing, where you focus on expanding your diaphragm and filling your lungs with air. By practicing diaphragmatic breathing regularly, you can strengthen your respiratory muscles and improve your lung capacity, which can help alleviate cough symptoms.

Another beneficial breathing exercise is pursed-lip breathing. This technique involves inhaling slowly through your nose and exhaling through pursed lips as if you are blowing out a candle. Pursed-lip breathing can help to regulate your breathing pattern, reduce shortness of breath, and calm coughing episodes.

To get the most out of breathing exercises, it is recommended to practice them regularly, preferably in a quiet and comfortable environment. Incorporating these exercises into your daily routine can provide long-term benefits for cough relief and respiratory health.

Salt Therapy

Salt therapy, also known as halotherapy, is a natural therapy that involves inhaling salt-infused air. It has been used for centuries to treat respiratory conditions and promote overall wellness. Salt therapy can be administered in various forms, such as salt caves, salt rooms, or salt inhalers.

The salt particles in the air during salt therapy are believed to have anti-inflammatory and antimicrobial properties. When inhaled, these particles can help to reduce inflammation in the airways, clear mucus, and kill bacteria or viruses that may be causing the cough.

Salt therapy can be particularly beneficial for individuals with respiratory conditions such as asthma, bronchitis, or allergies, which can often be accompanied by a persistent cough. By providing a natural and drug-free approach to cough relief, salt therapy can be a valuable addition to your cough management routine.

It is important to note that salt therapy may not be suitable for everyone, especially those with certain medical conditions or allergies. It is advisable to consult with a healthcare professional before trying salt therapy, especially if you have any concerns or underlying health issues.

Herbal Steam Inhalation

Herbal steam inhalation is a simple and effective alternative therapy for cough relief. It involves inhaling steam infused with medicinal herbs to soothe the respiratory system and alleviate cough symptoms.

To perform herbal steam inhalation, you can boil water in a pot and add a handful of dried herbs such as eucalyptus, thyme, or peppermint. Once the water is boiling, remove it from the heat and place a towel over your head, creating a tent-like structure to trap the steam. Lean over the pot, keeping a safe distance to avoid burns, and inhale the steam for about 10–15 minutes.

The steam helps to moisturize and soothe the airways, while the medicinal properties of the herbs provide additional relief.

Eucalyptus, for example, has expectorant properties that can help to loosen mucus and ease congestion. Thyme is known for its antimicrobial properties, which can help fight off respiratory infections. Peppermint has a cooling effect and can help to calm cough-related throat irritation.

Herbal steam inhalation can be performed once or twice a day, depending on the severity of your cough symptoms. It is a natural and gentle therapy that can provide immediate relief and promote respiratory health.

Chapter 3

Lifestyle Changes to Support Healing

Dietary Changes to Alleviate Cough Symptoms

When it comes to alleviating cough symptoms, many people overlook the role that diet plays in supporting the healing process. What we eat can have a significant impact on our respiratory health and the severity of our cough. In this section, we will explore some dietary changes that can help soothe and heal cough symptoms.

1. Stay hydrated.

One of the most important dietary changes you can make to alleviate cough symptoms is to stay hydrated. Drinking plenty of fluids helps to thin mucus and soothe the throat, making it easier to cough up phlegm. Water is the best choice, but herbal teas, warm broths, and soups can also provide hydration while offering additional benefits.

2. Include foods rich in vitamin C.

Vitamin C is known for its immune-boosting properties and its ability to reduce the duration and severity of respiratory infections. Including foods rich in vitamin C in your diet can help support your immune system and alleviate cough symptoms. Citrus fruits like oranges, lemons, and grapefruits are excellent sources of vitamin C. Other fruits and vegetables, such as strawberries, kiwi, bell peppers, and broccoli, are also high in this essential nutrient.

3. Incorporate anti-inflammatory foods.

Inflammation in the respiratory system can worsen cough symptoms. Including anti-inflammatory foods in your diet can help reduce inflammation and soothe the airways. Some examples of anti-inflammatory foods include fatty fish like salmon and sardines, nuts and seeds, olive oil, turmeric, ginger, and leafy green vegetables like spinach and kale.

4. Avoid irritants and allergens.

Certain foods can trigger or worsen cough symptoms, especially if you have allergies or sensitivities. It is important to identify and avoid these irritants and allergens to alleviate cough symptoms. Common culprits include dairy products, gluten, processed foods, and foods high in histamine, such as aged cheeses, fermented foods, and cured meats. Keeping a food diary can help you identify any potential triggers and make necessary dietary changes.

5. Include foods with natural cough-suppressing properties.

Some foods have natural cough-suppressing properties that can provide relief from persistent coughing. Including these foods in your diet can help soothe the throat and reduce coughing episodes. Honey is a well-known natural cough suppressant and can be added to warm herbal teas or consumed on its own. Other foods with cough-suppressing properties include pineapple, ginger, garlic, and licorice root.

6. Option for warm and soothing foods.

When you have a cough, opting for warm and soothing foods can provide comfort and relief. Warm liquids like herbal teas, warm broths, and soups can help soothe the throat and reduce coughing. Adding ingredients like ginger, turmeric, and garlic to your soups can provide additional anti-inflammatory and immune-boosting benefits. Avoiding cold and spicy foods can also help prevent further irritation of the throat and airways.

7. Consider probiotic-rich foods.

Probiotics are beneficial bacteria that can support a healthy immune system and improve respiratory health. Including probiotic-rich foods in your diet can help alleviate cough symptoms and promote healing. Yogurt, kefir, sauerkraut, kimchi, and other fermented foods are excellent sources of probiotics. Adding these foods to your diet can help maintain a healthy balance of bacteria in your gut and support your overall respiratory health.

8. Limit or avoid certain foods and beverages.

While there are foods that can help alleviate cough symptoms, there are also foods and beverages that can worsen them. It is important to limit or avoid these items to support the healing process. Some common culprits include caffeine, alcohol, sugary foods and beverages, and foods high in saturated fats. These substances can irritate the throat and airways, making cough symptoms more severe.

By making these dietary changes, you can support your body's natural healing process and alleviate cough symptoms. Remember to stay hydrated, include foods rich in vitamin C and anti-inflammatory properties, avoid irritants and allergens, incorporate foods with natural cough-suppressing properties, opt for warm and soothing foods, consider probiotic-rich foods, and limit or avoid certain foods and beverages. These dietary changes, combined with other natural remedies and lifestyle adjustments, can help you find relief from coughs and promote overall respiratory health.

Hydration and its Role in Cough Relief

When it comes to finding relief from a cough, one of the simplest and most effective remedies is often overlooked: hydration. Staying properly hydrated is essential for overall health, and it plays a crucial role in soothing and healing a cough.

When you have a cough, whether it's dry or productive, your respiratory system can become irritated and inflamed. This can lead to increased mucus production and a buildup of phlegm in your throat and lungs. By staying hydrated, you can help thin out the mucus and make it easier to expel, providing much-needed relief.

So, how does hydration help with cough relief? Let's take a closer look at the role it plays in soothing and healing your respiratory system.

The Importance of Drinking Water

Water is the foundation of hydration, and it should be your go-to beverage when you're dealing with a cough. Drinking an adequate amount of water throughout the day helps keep your respiratory system moist and hydrated. This can help soothe the irritated tissues in your throat and lungs, reducing coughing fits and discomfort.

When you're dehydrated, the mucus in your respiratory system becomes thicker and stickier. This can make it more difficult for your body to expel the mucus, leading to a persistent cough. By drinking enough water, you can help thin out the mucus, making it easier to cough up and clear your airways.

Herbal Teas for Hydration and Cough Relief

In addition to water, herbal teas can be a great way to stay hydrated and provide additional benefits for cough relief. Certain herbal teas, such as chamomile, ginger, and peppermint, have soothing properties that can help calm an irritated throat and reduce coughing.

Chamomile tea, in particular, has been used for centuries as a natural remedy for coughs and respiratory issues. It has anti-inflammatory properties that can help reduce swelling in the throat and soothe coughing spasms. Ginger tea is known for its warming and soothing effects, which can help alleviate cough symptoms. Peppermint tea has a cooling effect and can help relieve throat irritation and coughing.

When preparing herbal teas, it's important to avoid adding excessive amounts of sugar or honey, as these can worsen cough symptoms. Instead, opt for natural sweeteners like stevia or enjoy the teas plain.

Other Hydrating Beverages

While water and herbal teas should be your primary sources of hydration, other beverages can help soothe and heal your cough. Warm liquids, such as broths and soups, can provide additional hydration while also helping to thin out mucus and relieve congestion.

Warm water with a squeeze of lemon can also be beneficial for cough relief. Lemon is rich in vitamin C, which can help boost your immune system and support the healing process. Additionally, the acidity of lemon can help break up mucus and reduce coughing.

It's important to note that certain beverages, such as caffeinated drinks and alcohol, can have a dehydrating effect on the body. These should be consumed in moderation or avoided altogether when you're dealing with a cough.

Tips for Staying Hydrated

To ensure you're staying properly hydrated and maximizing the benefits of cough relief, here are some tips to keep in mind:

1. Drink water regularly throughout the day, aiming for at least 8 glasses (64 ounces) of water.

2. Keep a water bottle with you at all times to encourage regular hydration.

3. Sip on herbal teas, such as chamomile, ginger, and peppermint, to provide additional hydration and cough relief.

4. Enjoy warm liquids like broths, soups, and warm water with lemon to soothe your throat and thin out mucus.

5. Limit or avoid caffeinated drinks and alcohol, as they can dehydrate the body.

By prioritizing hydration and incorporating these tips into your daily routine, you can support your body's natural healing process and find relief from your cough more quickly.

Remember, staying hydrated is not only important for cough relief but also for overall respiratory health. By maintaining proper hydration, you can help prevent future coughs and respiratory issues. So, drink up and cough no more!

The Importance of Rest and Sleep in Healing

Rest and sleep are essential components of the healing process when it comes to cough relief. While it may seem counterintuitive, taking the time to rest and ensuring you get enough sleep can help speed up your recovery and alleviate cough symptoms. In this section, we will explore why rest and sleep are crucial for healing and provide some tips on how to optimize your rest and sleep to support your body's natural healing mechanisms.

The role of rest in healing

Rest is a fundamental aspect of the body's healing process. When you are sick with a cough, your body is working hard to fight off the underlying cause of the cough, whether it be a viral or bacterial infection, allergies, or other respiratory issues. By resting, you allow your body to conserve energy and redirect it towards the healing process.

During rest, your body can focus on repairing damaged tissues, strengthening the immune system, and reducing inflammation. It also helps to reduce stress on the body, which can further support the healing process. By giving yourself time and space to rest, you are giving your body the best chance to recover and heal from the cough.

The importance of sleep in healing

Sleep is a vital component of overall health and well-being, and it plays a crucial role in the healing process. When you sleep, your body goes through various stages of sleep, each with its unique functions. These stages include deep sleep and REM (rapid eye movement) sleep.

During deep sleep, your body releases growth hormones that help repair and regenerate tissues. This is particularly important when it comes to healing from a cough, as it allows your body to repair any damage to the respiratory system and strengthen the immune response. Deep sleep also plays a role in memory consolidation and cognitive function, which can be impaired when you are sleep-deprived.

REM sleep, on the other hand, is essential for brain function and emotional well-being. It is during this stage that your brain processes emotions and consolidates memories. Getting enough REM sleep can help reduce stress and anxiety, which can be beneficial for overall healing and cough relief.

Tips for optimizing rest and sleep

To ensure you are getting the rest and sleep you need to support your healing process, consider the following tips:

1. **Create a sleep-friendly environment:** Make sure your bedroom is cool, dark, and quiet. Use blackout curtains or an eye mask to block out any light, and consider using earplugs or a white noise machine to drown out any disruptive noises.

2. **Establish a bedtime routine:** Establishing a consistent bedtime routine can signal to your body that it's time to wind down and prepare for sleep. This can

include activities such as reading a book, taking a warm bath, or practicing relaxation techniques like deep breathing or meditation.

3. **Limit exposure to electronic devices:** The blue light emitted by electronic devices such as smartphones, tablets, and computers can interfere with your body's natural sleep-wake cycle. Try to limit your exposure to these devices at least an hour before bedtime to promote better sleep.

4. **Avoid caffeine and stimulants:** Caffeine and other stimulants can interfere with your ability to fall asleep and stay asleep. Avoid consuming caffeine-containing beverages or foods, such as coffee, tea, chocolate, and energy drinks, in the evening.

5. **Practice good sleep hygiene:** Establishing good sleep hygiene habits can help improve the quality of your sleep. This includes going to bed and waking up at the same time every day, avoiding naps during the day, and creating a comfortable sleep environment.

6. **Manage stress:** Stress can disrupt sleep and hinder the healing process. Find healthy ways to manage stress, such as engaging in relaxation techniques, practicing mindfulness or yoga, or seeking support from a therapist or counselor.

7. **Listen to your body:** Pay attention to your body's signals, and permit yourself to rest when you need it. Pushing yourself too hard can prolong the healing process and make your cough symptoms worse.

Remember, rest and sleep are not signs of weakness but rather essential components of the healing process. By prioritizing rest and ensuring you get enough sleep, you are giving your body the best chance to recover and heal from a cough. So, make it a priority to create a sleep-friendly environment, establish a bedtime routine, and practice good sleep hygiene. Your body will thank you for it.

Managing Stress and its Impact on Cough

Stress is a common factor in our daily lives, and it can have a significant impact on our overall health and well-being. When it comes to coughing, stress can exacerbate symptoms and make it more difficult for our bodies to heal. In this section, we will explore the relationship between stress and coughing and discuss strategies for managing stress to promote cough relief and healing.

The Link Between Stress and Cough

Stress affects our bodies in various ways, and one of the ways it can manifest is through coughing. When we are stressed, our bodies release stress hormones, such as cortisol, which can suppress our immune system and increase inflammation in our respiratory system. This can make us more susceptible to respiratory infections and irritate our airways, leading to coughing.

Furthermore, stress can also contribute to the development of a chronic cough. Chronic cough is defined as a cough that lasts for more than eight weeks and is often associated with underlying medical conditions such as asthma, allergies, or acid reflux. Stress can worsen these conditions and trigger or prolong coughing episodes.

Stress Management Techniques for Cough Relief

Managing stress is crucial not only for our overall well-being but also for alleviating cough symptoms and promoting healing. Here are some effective stress management techniques that can help reduce coughing:

1. **Deep Breathing and Relaxation Exercises:** Deep breathing exercises, such as diaphragmatic breathing, can help calm our nervous system and reduce stress levels. Find a quiet and comfortable place to sit or lie down, close your eyes, and take slow, deep breaths. Focus on filling your abdomen with air as you inhale and slowly exhale. This simple technique can help

relax your body and mind, reducing stress and potentially alleviating coughing.

2. **Meditation and Mindfulness:** Practicing meditation and mindfulness can be powerful tools for managing stress and promoting relaxation. Find a quiet space, sit comfortably, and focus your attention on your breath or a specific object. Allow your thoughts to come and go without judgment. By practicing mindfulness regularly, you can train your mind to stay present and reduce stress levels, which may have a positive impact on your cough symptoms.

3. **Exercise and Physical Activity:** Engaging in regular exercise and physical activity can help reduce stress and improve overall well-being. Exercise releases endorphins, which are natural mood boosters, and can help distract your mind from stressors. Choose activities that you enjoy, such as walking, jogging, yoga, or dancing, and aim for at least 30 minutes of moderate-intensity exercise most days of the week. Not only will exercise help manage stress, but it can also improve your respiratory health and support the healing process.

4. **Relaxation Techniques:** Incorporating relaxation techniques into your daily routine can help reduce

stress and promote cough relief. Consider trying techniques such as progressive muscle relaxation, where you systematically tense and relax different muscle groups, or guided imagery, where you visualize calming and peaceful scenes. Experiment with different relaxation techniques to find what works best for you and make it a regular part of your stress management routine.

5. **Social Support and Connection:** Maintaining social connections and seeking support from loved ones can be instrumental in managing stress. Share your concerns and feelings with trusted friends or family members, or consider joining a support group where you can connect with others who may be experiencing similar challenges. Having a strong support network can provide emotional support, reduce feelings of isolation, and help alleviate stress, which may positively impact your cough symptoms.

Creating a Stress-Reducing Environment

In addition to practicing stress management techniques, creating a stress-reducing environment can also contribute to cough relief and healing. Here are some tips for creating a calming and supportive environment:

1. Declutter your living space to create a sense of calm and order.
2. Use soothing colors and lighting in your home to promote relaxation.
3. Incorporate calming scents, such as lavender or chamomile, through essential oils or candles.
4. Create a bedtime routine that promotes restful sleep, such as reading a book or taking a warm bath.
5. Limit exposure to stressful situations or triggers, such as excessive noise or negative news.

By implementing these strategies and creating a stress-reducing environment, you can help manage stress levels, reduce coughing episodes, and support your body's natural healing process.

Remember, managing stress is a lifelong practice, and it may take time to find the techniques that work best for you. Be patient with yourself and prioritize self-care to promote overall well-being and alleviate cough symptoms.

Chapter 4

Natural Remedies for Specific Types of Cough

Remedies for Dry Cough

A dry cough can be irritating and uncomfortable, often causing a tickling or scratching sensation in the throat. It is important to address a dry cough promptly to prevent it from worsening or becoming chronic. In this section, we will explore various natural remedies that can help soothe and heal a dry cough.

1. **Honey and Warm Water:** One of the simplest and most effective remedies for a dry cough is a mixture of honey and warm water. Honey contains natural soothing properties that can help relieve throat irritation. Drink a glass of warm water slowly after adding one to two tablespoons of honey to it. You can also add a squeeze of lemon juice for added benefits. This remedy can be repeated several times a day, as needed.

2. **Steam Inhalation:** Steam inhalation is a great way to relieve a dry cough and clear congestion in the respiratory tract. Add a few drops of peppermint or eucalyptus essential oils to a bowl of hot water. Lean over the bowl, wrap a towel around your head to trap the steam, and inhale deeply for about 10 minutes. The steam helps to moisturize the airways and reduce irritation, providing relief from a dry cough.

3. **Ginger Tea:** Ginger has long been used for its medicinal properties, which include the ability to relieve coughs and reduce inflammation. To make ginger tea, grate a small piece of fresh ginger and steep it in hot water for 10 minutes. Honey and lemon juice can be added for extra flavor and health benefits. To help relieve a dry cough, drink this tea two to three times per day.

4. **Marshmallow Root:** Marshmallow root is a herb that has been used for centuries to soothe coughs and sore throats. It contains mucilage, a substance that forms a protective layer in the throat, reducing irritation and promoting healing. You can make marshmallow root tea by steeping one teaspoon of dried marshmallow root in a cup of hot water for 10 minutes. Strain the tea

and drink it warm. This remedy can be repeated several times a day, as needed.

5. **Licorice Root:** Licorice root is another herb that can help soothe a dry cough. It has expectorant properties, which means it helps to loosen and expel mucus from the respiratory tract. Licorice root also has anti-inflammatory properties that can reduce irritation in the throat. You can make licorice root tea by steeping one teaspoon of dried licorice root in a cup of hot water for 10 minutes. Strain the tea and drink it warm. It is important to remember that licorice root should only be consumed in moderation and should not be consumed by people with high blood pressure.

6. **Thyme Infusion:** Thyme is a herb that has been used for centuries for its medicinal properties. It contains compounds that have antitussive (cough-suppressing) and expectorant properties, making it an excellent remedy for a dry cough. To make a thyme infusion, steep one teaspoon of dried thyme leaves in a cup of hot water for 10 minutes. Strain the infusion and drink it warm. You can add honey or lemon juice for added flavor and benefits. This remedy can be repeated several times a day, as needed.

7. **Saltwater Gargle:** Gargling with salt water can help soothe a dry cough by reducing inflammation and irritation in the throat. Mix half a teaspoon of salt in a glass of warm water and stir until the salt is dissolved. Gargle with this solution for 30 seconds, then spit it out. Repeat this process several times a day to help alleviate a dry cough.

8. **Slippery Elm Bark:** Slippery elm bark is a natural remedy that can help soothe a dry cough and reduce throat irritation. It contains mucilage, which forms a protective layer in the throat, providing relief from coughing. You can make slippery elm bark tea by steeping one teaspoon of powdered slippery elm bark in a cup of hot water for 10 minutes. Strain the tea and drink it warm. This remedy can be repeated several times a day, as needed.

9. **Turmeric Milk:** Turmeric is a spice that has been used for its medicinal properties for centuries. It contains curcumin, a compound with anti-inflammatory and antioxidant properties. Turmeric milk is a popular remedy for a dry cough, as it helps to reduce inflammation in the respiratory tract and soothe irritation. To make turmeric milk, heat a cup of milk and add half a teaspoon of turmeric powder. You can

also add a pinch of black pepper for better absorption. Drink this mixture before bedtime to help alleviate a dry cough.

10. **Probiotics:** Probiotics are beneficial bacteria that can help support a healthy immune system and reduce the severity and duration of a cough. They can be found in fermented foods such as yogurt, kefir, sauerkraut, and kimchi. Including these probiotic-rich foods in your diet can help promote respiratory health and alleviate a dry cough.

These natural remedies can provide relief from a dry cough and promote healing. If your cough lasts longer than two weeks or is accompanied by other severe symptoms, you should seek medical attention. Remember to consult with a healthcare professional before trying any new remedies, especially if you have any underlying health conditions or are taking medications.

Remedies for a Wet or Productive Cough

A wet or productive cough is characterized by the presence of mucus or phlegm. It is often a sign that your body is trying to clear out excess mucus or irritants from your respiratory system. While it can be uncomfortable and disruptive, several natural remedies can help soothe and alleviate a wet cough.

1. **Stay Hydrated:** One of the most important remedies for a wet cough is to stay hydrated. Drinking plenty of fluids helps to thin the mucus, making it easier to expel from your body. Drink at least 8-10 glasses of water per day. You can also try warm liquids like herbal teas, broths, or warm water with honey and lemon, which can help soothe your throat and provide relief.

2. **Steam Inhalation:** Steam inhalation is a simple yet effective remedy for a wet cough. The warm, moist air helps to loosen the mucus in your airways, making it easier to cough up. You can do this by filling a bowl with hot water and leaning over it, covering your head with a towel to trap the steam. Breathe deeply for about 10 minutes, keeping a safe distance from the hot water to avoid burns.

3. **Saltwater Gargle:** Gargling with warm salt water can help soothe a sore throat and reduce the severity of a wet cough. In a glass of warm water, dissolve half a teaspoon of salt and gargle for 30 seconds before spitting it out. Repeat several times per day to help reduce throat inflammation and irritation.

4. **Honey and Ginger:** Both honey and ginger have natural antibacterial and anti-inflammatory properties that can help alleviate a wet cough. Mix one

tablespoon of honey with a few drops of fresh ginger juice and consume it two to three times a day. Alternatively, you can add ginger slices to a cup of boiling water, let it steep for 10 minutes, strain, and then add honey to taste. Drink this ginger tea two to three times a day for relief.

5. **Herbal Expectorants:** Certain herbs have expectorant properties, meaning they help to loosen and expel mucus from the respiratory system. Some commonly used herbs for wet coughs include licorice root, marshmallow root, and mullein. You can find these herbs in the form of teas, tinctures, or capsules at health food stores. Follow the instructions on the packaging for proper dosage and usage.

6. **Eucalyptus Oil:** Eucalyptus oil is known for its decongestant and expectorant properties, making it an excellent remedy for a wet cough. You can add a few drops of eucalyptus oil to a bowl of hot water and inhale the steam, or you can mix it with a carrier oil like coconut oil and apply it to your chest and throat for relief. Remember to perform a patch test before applying it to your skin to ensure you are not allergic to it.

7. **Onion Syrup:** Onions have natural antimicrobial properties and can help soothe a wet cough. To make onion syrup, chop a medium-sized onion and place it in a bowl. Add enough honey to cover the onion, and let it sit overnight. The next day, strain the mixture and take one tablespoon of the syrup every few hours to help alleviate your cough.

8. **Warm Compress:** Applying a warm compress to your chest and back can help relieve congestion and loosen mucus, providing relief from a wet cough. Soak a clean towel in warm water, wring out the excess, and place it on your chest and back for 10–15 minutes. Repeat this several times a day as needed.

9. **Avoid Irritants:** To prevent further irritation and exacerbation of your wet cough, it is important to avoid irritants such as smoke, dust, and strong chemical fumes. These can further irritate your respiratory system and make your cough worse. If possible, stay in a clean and well-ventilated environment and avoid exposure to these irritants.

10. **Relaxation:** Resting and allowing your body to heal is crucial when dealing with a wet cough. Adequate rest helps boost your immune system and allows your body to focus on fighting off the infection or irritants

causing the cough. Make sure to get enough sleep and take breaks throughout the day to relax and reduce stress, as stress can weaken your immune system and prolong your cough.

Remember, while these natural remedies can provide relief for a wet cough, it is important to consult with a healthcare professional if your symptoms persist or worsen. They can help determine the underlying cause of your cough and provide appropriate treatment if necessary.

Remedies for Persistent or Chronic Cough

A persistent or chronic cough can be frustrating and disruptive to your daily life. It is important to address the underlying cause of the cough to find relief. In this section, we will explore natural remedies that can help soothe and heal a persistent or chronic cough.

1. **Honey and Lemon:** One of the most effective remedies for a persistent or chronic cough is a combination of honey and lemon. Honey has natural antibacterial properties and can help soothe the throat, while lemon provides vitamin C and antioxidants to boost the immune system. Mix one tablespoon of honey with the juice of half a lemon in a cup of warm

water. To help relieve your cough, drink this mixture several times per day.

2. **Ginger Tea:** Ginger has long been used as a natural cough and cold remedy. It has anti-inflammatory properties that can help relieve irritation in the throat and airways. Grate some fresh ginger and steep it in hot water for ten minutes to make ginger tea. Add honey and lemon for additional benefits. To help with your persistent cough, consume this tea two to three times daily.

3. **Steam Inhalation:** Steam inhalation is a simple and effective method for relieving a persistent cough. The steam moisturizes and soothes the airways, reducing irritation and promoting healing. Bring a pot of water to a boil, then carefully place your face over the steam, covering your head with a towel to trap the steam. Breathe deeply for 10 to 15 minutes. For extra benefits, add a few drops of essential oils like eucalyptus or peppermint.

4. **Marshmallow Root:** Marshmallow root has been used for centuries to soothe coughs and sore throats. It contains mucilage, a substance that forms a protective layer in the throat, reducing irritation and promoting healing. You can make marshmallow root tea by

steeping one tablespoon of dried marshmallow root in a cup of hot water for 10–15 minutes. Strain and drink this tea two to three times a day to help alleviate your persistent cough.

5. **Licorice Root:** Licorice root is another natural remedy that can help soothe a persistent cough. It has expectorant properties, which means it helps to loosen and expel mucus from the airways. Licorice root also has anti-inflammatory properties that can reduce irritation in the throat. You can make licorice root tea by steeping one teaspoon of dried licorice root in a cup of hot water for 10 minutes. Drink this tea two to three times a day to help relieve your cough.

6. **Turmeric Milk:** Turmeric is a powerful anti-inflammatory spice that can help reduce inflammation in the airways and soothe a persistent cough. Mix one teaspoon of turmeric powder with a cup of warm milk. You can also add a pinch of black pepper to enhance the absorption of turmeric. Drink this mixture before bedtime to help alleviate your cough and promote restful sleep.

7. **Saltwater Gargle:** Gargling with saltwater can help soothe a persistent cough by reducing inflammation and irritation in the throat. Mix half a teaspoon of salt

in a glass of warm water and gargle for 30 seconds, then spit it out. Repeat this several times a day to help relieve your cough.

8. **Probiotics:** Probiotics are beneficial bacteria that can help support a healthy immune system and reduce cough symptoms. They can be found in fermented foods such as yogurt, kefir, sauerkraut, and kimchi. Incorporate these foods into your diet to help alleviate your persistent cough.

9. **Breathing Exercises:** Certain breathing exercises can help strengthen the respiratory muscles and improve lung function, which can in turn reduce cough symptoms. One simple exercise is diaphragmatic breathing, where you focus on breathing deeply into your diaphragm rather than shallowly into your chest. Practice this exercise for a few minutes each day to help alleviate your persistent cough.

10. **Avoid Irritants:** If you have a persistent cough, it is important to avoid irritants that can worsen your symptoms. This includes cigarette smoke, air pollution, strong perfumes, and cleaning products with strong fumes. By minimizing exposure to these irritants, you can help reduce the frequency and severity of your cough.

Remember, while these natural remedies can provide relief for a persistent or chronic cough, it is important to consult with a healthcare professional if your symptoms persist or worsen. They can help determine the underlying cause of your cough and provide appropriate treatment options.

Remedies for Coughs Associated with Allergies

Allergies can be a major trigger for coughing in adults. When your body comes into contact with an allergen, such as pollen, dust mites, or pet dander, it can cause an allergic reaction that leads to coughing. This cough is often accompanied by sneezing, itching, and a runny nose. If caused by allergies, natural remedies can bring relief.

1. **Identify and Avoid Allergens:** The first step in managing a cough associated with allergies is to identify and avoid the allergens that trigger your symptoms. Keep a diary of when your cough worsens and try to pinpoint any patterns or triggers. Common allergens include pollen, mold, dust mites, pet dander, and certain foods. Once you've identified your triggers, take steps to minimize your exposure to them. For example, if pollen is a trigger, try to stay indoors on high pollen days or use an air purifier in your home.

2. **Nasal Irrigation:** Nasal irrigation can help relieve allergy-related coughs by flushing out irritants and reducing inflammation in the nasal passages. You can use a neti pot or a saline nasal spray to rinse your nasal passages with a saltwater solution. This can help remove allergens and mucus, providing relief from coughing and congestion. Make sure to use distilled or sterile water and follow the instructions carefully to avoid any complications.

3. **Honey:** Honey has long been used as a natural remedy for cough and throat irritation. It has soothing properties that can help alleviate coughing caused by allergies. You can mix a teaspoon of honey with warm water or herbal tea and drink it several times a day. However, it's important to note that honey should not be given to children under the age of one due to the risk of botulism.

4. **Steam Inhalation:** Steam inhalation can provide temporary relief from coughing associated with allergies. The warm, moist air can help soothe irritated airways and loosen mucus. You can simply fill a bowl with hot water, place a towel over your head, and inhale the steam for a few minutes. Adding a few drops of essential oils like eucalyptus or peppermint can

enhance the benefits. However, be cautious with steam inhalation if you have asthma, as it can trigger symptoms in some individuals.

5. **Quercetin-Rich Foods:** Quercetin is a natural compound found in certain foods that has anti-inflammatory and antihistamine properties. Consuming foods rich in quercetin can help reduce allergic reactions and alleviate coughing. Some quercetin-rich foods include apples, berries, onions, citrus fruits, broccoli, and leafy greens. Incorporate these foods into your diet to support your body's natural defense against allergies.

6. **Probiotics:** Probiotics are beneficial bacteria that can help regulate the immune system and reduce allergic reactions. They can be particularly helpful in managing coughs associated with allergies. You can find probiotics in fermented foods like yogurt, kefir, sauerkraut, and kimchi. Alternatively, you can take probiotic supplements, but it's always best to consult with a healthcare professional before starting any new supplement regimen.

7. **Vitamin C:** Vitamin C can boost immunity, reduce inflammation, and ease coughing from allergies. Incorporate vitamin C-rich foods into your diet, such

as citrus fruits, strawberries, kiwi, bell peppers, and leafy greens. You can also consider taking a vitamin C supplement, but it's important to follow the recommended dosage and consult with a healthcare professional if you have any underlying health conditions.

8. **Herbal Teas:** Certain herbal teas can provide relief from coughing associated with allergies. Chamomile tea has anti-inflammatory properties and can help soothe irritated airways. Peppermint tea has a cooling effect and can help alleviate coughing and congestion. Licorice root tea can help reduce inflammation and soothe the throat. Drink these teas warm and inhale the steam for added benefits.

9. **Acupuncture:** Acupuncture is an alternative therapy that involves the insertion of thin needles into specific points of the body. It has been used for centuries to treat various health conditions, including allergies and coughing. Acupuncture may help regulate the immune system and reduce inflammation, providing relief from allergy-related coughing. Consult with a licensed acupuncturist to determine if this therapy is suitable for you.

10. **Air Purification:** Investing in an air purifier can help remove allergens from the air and improve indoor air quality. Look for an air purifier with a HEPA filter, as it can effectively capture small particles like pollen, dust mites, and pet dander. Place the air purifier in your bedroom or any other room where you spend a significant amount of time to reduce your exposure to allergens and minimize coughing.

Remember, while these natural remedies can provide relief from coughing associated with allergies, it's important to consult with a healthcare professional if your symptoms persist or worsen. They can help determine the underlying cause of your cough and provide appropriate treatment options.

Chapter 5

Caring for Your Respiratory Health

Maintaining a Healthy Lifestyle for Respiratory Health

Maintaining a healthy lifestyle is crucial for overall well-being, and it plays a significant role in supporting respiratory health. By adopting certain habits and making conscious choices, you can strengthen your respiratory system and reduce the risk of respiratory issues. In this section, we will explore some key aspects of a healthy lifestyle that can contribute to optimal respiratory health.

1. Nourishing your body with a balanced diet

A balanced diet is essential for maintaining respiratory health. Including a variety of nutrient-rich foods can provide your body with the necessary vitamins and minerals to support lung function. Focus on incorporating foods that are known to have anti-inflammatory properties, such as fruits, vegetables, whole grains, and lean proteins. These foods can help reduce inflammation in the airways and promote healthy lung function.

Additionally, certain nutrients are particularly beneficial for respiratory health. Omega-3 fatty acids, found in fatty fish like salmon and sardines, have anti-inflammatory properties and may help reduce the risk of respiratory conditions. Vitamin C, found in citrus fruits and leafy greens, can strengthen the immune system and protect against respiratory infections. Foods rich in antioxidants, such as berries and green tea, can also support respiratory health by reducing oxidative stress in the body.

2. Staying active and exercising regularly

Regular physical activity is not only beneficial for cardiovascular health but also plays a crucial role in maintaining respiratory health. Engaging in aerobic exercises, such as brisk walking, jogging, or cycling, can improve lung capacity and strengthen the respiratory muscles. These exercises increase the oxygen demand, which helps train the lungs to work more efficiently.

In addition to aerobic exercises, incorporating specific exercises that target the respiratory muscles can further enhance lung function. Deep breathing exercises, such as diaphragmatic breathing and pursed-lip breathing, can help improve lung capacity and promote better oxygen exchange. These exercises can be particularly beneficial for individuals with respiratory conditions such as asthma or chronic obstructive pulmonary disease (COPD).

3. Avoiding exposure to respiratory irritants

Reducing exposure to respiratory irritants is crucial for maintaining respiratory health. Environmental factors such as air pollution, secondhand smoke, and chemical fumes can irritate the airways and increase the risk of respiratory issues. Whenever possible, try to avoid or minimize exposure to these irritants.

If you live in an area with high levels of air pollution, consider using air purifiers in your home to filter out harmful particles. When outdoors, try to avoid heavily trafficked areas and stay indoors during times of high pollution. If you are a smoker, quitting smoking is one of the best things you can do for your respiratory health. Secondhand smoke is equally harmful, so it's important to avoid exposure to smoke from others as well.

4. Maintaining a healthy weight

Maintaining a healthy weight is not only important for overall health but also for respiratory health. Excess weight can put pressure on the lungs and diaphragm, making it harder to breathe efficiently. It can also increase the risk of developing respiratory conditions such as asthma or sleep apnea.

If you are overweight or obese, losing weight through a combination of a balanced diet and regular exercise can significantly improve respiratory function. Consult with a healthcare professional or a registered dietitian to develop a personalized weight loss plan that suits your needs and goals.

5. Practicing good hygiene and preventing infections

Practicing good hygiene is essential for preventing respiratory infections and maintaining respiratory health. Wash your hands frequently with soap and water, especially before eating or touching your face. Avoid close contact with individuals who have respiratory infections, such as the common cold or the flu.

In addition to good hygiene practices, getting vaccinated against respiratory infections can provide an extra layer of protection. Annual flu shots are recommended for everyone, particularly individuals with respiratory conditions or weakened immune systems. Vaccines for other respiratory infections, such as pneumonia, may also be recommended based on your age and overall health.

6. Managing stress and promoting relaxation

Chronic stress can hurt respiratory health. When you are stressed, your body releases stress hormones that can affect the immune system and increase inflammation in the airways.

Finding healthy ways to manage stress and promote relaxation can help support respiratory health.

Engaging in activities such as yoga, meditation, or deep breathing exercises can help reduce stress levels and promote a sense of calm. Prioritizing self-care and taking time for activities that bring you joy and relaxation can also contribute to overall well-being, including respiratory health.

By incorporating these lifestyle habits into your daily routine, you can support and maintain optimal respiratory health. Remember, small changes can make a big difference, so start implementing these habits gradually and consistently for long-term benefits.

Exercises and Techniques to Improve Lung Function

When it comes to caring for your respiratory health, it's not just about finding remedies for cough relief. It's also important to focus on improving your lung function. By incorporating specific exercises and techniques into your daily routine, you can strengthen your respiratory muscles and enhance your lung capacity. In this section, we will explore various exercises and techniques that can help improve your lung function.

1. Deep Breathing Exercises

Improving lung function can be simple yet effective with deep breathing exercises. These exercises can expand your lung capacity and increase the amount of oxygen you take in with each breath. Here are a few examples of deep breathing exercises you can try:

- **Diaphragmatic Breathing:** Sit or lie down in a comfortable position. Place one hand on your chest and the other on your abdomen. Take a slow, deep breath in through your nose, allowing your abdomen to rise as you fill your lungs with air. Exhale slowly through your mouth, feeling your abdomen fall. Repeat this exercise for several minutes, focusing on deep, slow breaths.

- **Pursed Lip Breathing:** Pursed lip breathing can help improve the efficiency of your breathing and reduce shortness of breath. Inhale slowly through your nose for a count of two. Then, purse your lips as if you were going to blow out a candle and exhale slowly for a count of four. Repeat this exercise for several minutes, gradually increasing the duration of your exhalation.

- **Segmental Breathing:** This exercise helps improve the movement of your ribcage and encourages deep breathing. Place your hands on the sides of your ribcage. Take a deep breath in, focusing on expanding the lower part of your ribcage. Exhale slowly, feeling your ribcage contract. Move your hands up to the middle of your ribcage and repeat the process. Finally, move your hands to the upper part of your ribcage and repeat the exercise. This exercise can be done while sitting or standing.

2. Aerobic Exercises

Engaging in regular aerobic exercises can have a positive impact on your lung function. These exercises increase your heart rate and breathing rate, helping to strengthen your respiratory muscles and improve your lung capacity. Here are a few aerobic exercises that can benefit your respiratory health:

- **Brisk Walking:** Walking is a low-impact aerobic exercise that can be easily incorporated into your daily routine. Aim for a brisk pace that elevates your heart rate and makes you slightly breathless. Start with shorter walks and gradually increase the duration and intensity over time.

- **Cycling:** Cycling is another excellent aerobic exercise that can help improve lung function. Whether you prefer outdoor cycling or using a stationary bike, this activity can strengthen your leg muscles and increase your lung capacity. Start with shorter cycling sessions and gradually increase the duration and intensity as your fitness improves.

- **Swimming:** Swimming is a highly beneficial exercise for respiratory health. The combination of aerobic activity and the humid environment of the pool can help improve lung function and reduce respiratory symptoms. If you're new to swimming, start with shorter sessions and gradually increase the duration as you build your stamina.

3. Breathing Techniques

In addition to deep breathing exercises, certain breathing techniques can also help improve lung function and alleviate respiratory symptoms. Here are a few techniques you can incorporate into your daily routine:

- **Paced Breathing:** Paced breathing involves consciously slowing down your breathing rate. Take slow, deep breaths in through your nose and exhale slowly through your mouth. Aim to extend the duration of your inhalation and exhalation, gradually working towards a ratio of 1:2 (inhale for a count of four, exhale for a count of eight). This technique can help relax your respiratory muscles and improve lung function.

- **Lip Flutters:** Lip flutters, also known as "blowing raspberries," can help strengthen your respiratory muscles. Pucker your lips and exhale forcefully, creating a fluttering sound. Repeat this exercise several times, gradually increasing the duration of each flutter. This technique can help improve lung capacity and enhance the control of your exhalation.

- **Incentive Spirometry:** Incentive spirometry is a device that can be used to improve lung function and prevent respiratory complications. It involves inhaling deeply through a mouthpiece, which raises a ball or piston in the device. This exercise helps expand your lung capacity and encourages deep breathing. Consult with a healthcare professional to learn how to use an incentive spirometer correctly.

By incorporating these exercises and techniques into your daily routine, you can improve your lung function and support your respiratory health. Remember to start slowly and gradually increase the intensity and duration of your exercises. If you have any underlying health conditions or concerns, it's always a good idea to consult with a healthcare professional before starting a new exercise regimen.

Preventing Respiratory Infections

Respiratory infections can be a major cause of coughing and discomfort. They can range from mild colds to more severe conditions like bronchitis or pneumonia. Preventing respiratory infections is crucial for maintaining respiratory health and avoiding the discomfort and inconvenience they bring. In this section, we will explore some effective strategies to help you prevent respiratory infections and keep your respiratory system in optimal condition.

1. Practice good hygiene

One of the most effective ways to prevent respiratory infections is by practicing good hygiene. This includes washing your hands frequently with soap and water for at least 20 seconds, especially before eating or touching your face. Hand sanitizers can be used when soap and water are not readily available. Avoid touching your face, particularly your eyes, nose, and mouth, as these are entry points for viruses and bacteria.

Covering your mouth and nose with a tissue or your elbow when coughing or sneezing can help prevent the spread of respiratory infections. Dispose of used tissues properly, and wash your hands afterward. If you don't have a tissue, cough or sneeze into your elbow rather than your hands to minimize the spread of germs.

2. Maintain a healthy lifestyle

A healthy lifestyle plays a significant role in preventing respiratory infections. Eating a balanced diet rich in fruits, vegetables, whole grains, and lean proteins can boost your immune system and help fight off infections. Include foods that are high in vitamins A, C, and E, as these are known to support respiratory health.

Regular exercise is also essential for maintaining a strong immune system. Engaging in moderate-intensity exercise for at least 30 minutes a day can improve blood circulation and enhance the function of your respiratory system. Additionally, getting enough sleep is crucial for a healthy immune system. Aim for 7-9 hours of quality sleep each night to support your body's natural defense mechanisms.

3. Avoid exposure to respiratory irritants

Exposure to respiratory irritants can weaken your respiratory system and make you more susceptible to infections. Avoid smoking and secondhand smoke, as they can damage the lining of your respiratory tract and impair your lung function. If you are a smoker, consider quitting to reduce your risk of respiratory infections and other respiratory diseases.

Air pollution can also be a significant respiratory irritant. Limit your exposure to outdoor air pollution by staying indoors on days with poor air quality or wearing a mask when necessary. Additionally, ensure good ventilation in your home to reduce indoor air pollution from sources such as cooking fumes, cleaning products, and mold.

4. Boost your immune system

A strong immune system is your body's first line of defense against respiratory infections. There are several ways you can boost your immune system naturally. Consuming foods rich in antioxidants, such as berries, citrus fruits, and leafy greens, can help strengthen your immune system. Probiotics, found in yogurt and fermented foods, can also support a healthy immune system.

Getting regular exercise, managing stress levels, and maintaining a healthy weight are all factors that contribute to a robust immune system. Engaging in stress-reducing activities like meditation, yoga, or deep breathing exercises can help lower your risk of respiratory infections. Additionally, maintaining a healthy weight can reduce the strain on your respiratory system and improve its overall function.

5. Stay up-to-date with vaccinations

Vaccinations are an essential tool for preventing respiratory infections. Make sure you are up to date with recommended vaccinations, such as the flu vaccine and the pneumonia vaccine. These vaccines can significantly reduce your risk of developing severe respiratory infections and their complications.

It is especially important for individuals at higher risk, such as older adults, young children, and those with chronic medical conditions, to receive vaccinations. Consult with your healthcare provider to determine which vaccinations are appropriate for you based on your age, health status, and any specific risk factors you may have.

6. Avoid close contact with sick individuals

Respiratory infections are often contagious and can spread through close contact with infected individuals. If someone around you is sick with a respiratory infection, try to maintain a safe distance and avoid close contact. This includes avoiding crowded places or gatherings where the risk of exposure to respiratory infections may be higher.

If you are the one who is sick, it is important to take precautions to prevent spreading the infection to others. Stay home from work or school, cover your mouth and nose when coughing or sneezing, and dispose of used tissues properly. By taking these simple steps, you can help protect those around you from respiratory infections.

7. Keep your environment clean

Maintaining a clean environment can help reduce the risk of respiratory infections. Regularly clean and disinfect frequently touched surfaces, such as doorknobs, light switches, and countertops. Pay special attention to areas where germs are more likely to accumulate, such as bathrooms and kitchens.

Properly ventilate your living spaces to ensure good air circulation. Use air purifiers or open windows to improve indoor air quality and reduce the concentration of airborne pathogens. Regularly change and clean the air filters in your heating and cooling systems to prevent the buildup of dust and allergens.

By following these preventive measures, you can significantly reduce your risk of respiratory infections and promote the overall health of your respiratory system. Remember, prevention is always better than cure when it comes to respiratory health.

When to Consult a Healthcare Professional for Respiratory Issues

While natural remedies can be effective in managing and alleviating cough symptoms, there are certain situations where it is important to seek medical attention for respiratory issues. It is crucial to recognize when self-care measures are not enough and when it is necessary to consult a healthcare professional. This section will guide you on when to seek medical help for respiratory issues and what signs to look out for.

1. Persistent or worsening symptoms

If you have been experiencing a cough that persists for more than three weeks or if your symptoms are getting worse despite trying various natural remedies, it is advisable to consult a healthcare professional. Persistent coughing can be a sign of an underlying condition that requires medical intervention. Your healthcare provider will be able to assess your symptoms, conduct a thorough examination, and recommend appropriate treatment options.

2. Difficulty breathing or shortness of breath

If you are experiencing difficulty breathing or shortness of breath along with your cough, it is essential to seek immediate medical attention. These symptoms could indicate a more serious respiratory condition, such as asthma, pneumonia, or chronic obstructive pulmonary disease (COPD). A healthcare professional will be able to evaluate your breathing patterns, perform necessary tests, and provide appropriate treatment to alleviate your symptoms and improve your respiratory health.

3. Chest pain or tightness

If your cough is accompanied by chest pain or tightness, it is important not to ignore these symptoms. Chest pain can be a sign of various respiratory conditions, including bronchitis, pneumonia, or even a heart-related issue. Seeking medical attention will allow a healthcare professional to evaluate your symptoms, conduct any necessary tests, and provide appropriate treatment to address the underlying cause of your discomfort.

4. Coughing up blood

Coughing up blood, also known as hemoptysis, is a serious symptom that should never be ignored. It can be a sign of a severe respiratory condition such as tuberculosis, lung cancer, or a pulmonary embolism. If you notice blood in your cough, it is crucial to seek immediate medical attention. A healthcare professional will be able to assess your condition, conduct diagnostic tests, and provide appropriate treatment to address the underlying cause of the bleeding.

5. High fever

If your cough is accompanied by a high fever, it may indicate an infection that requires medical attention. A persistent high fever can be a sign of pneumonia or other respiratory infections. It is important to consult a healthcare professional who can evaluate your symptoms, perform necessary tests, and prescribe appropriate medications to treat the infection and alleviate your cough.

6. Respiratory issues in children or older adults

If a child or an older adult is experiencing respiratory issues, it is advisable to consult a healthcare professional. Children and older adults may be more vulnerable to respiratory infections and may require specialized care. A healthcare professional will be able to assess the severity of the symptoms, provide appropriate treatment options, and monitor the individual's respiratory health closely.

7. Underlying health conditions

If you have pre-existing health conditions such as asthma, COPD, or any other chronic respiratory condition, it is important to consult a healthcare professional for any new or worsening symptoms. These conditions may require specific management strategies and medications that can only be prescribed by a healthcare professional. Regular check-ups and consultations with your healthcare provider are essential to ensuring optimal respiratory health.

8. Concerns about medication interactions

If you are currently taking any medications for other health conditions and are unsure about potential interactions with natural remedies or over-the-counter cough medications, it is best to consult a healthcare professional. They will be able to review your medication regimen, guide potential interactions, and suggest alternative remedies or treatments that are safe and effective for your specific situation.

Remember, while natural remedies can be beneficial in managing cough symptoms, it is important to seek medical attention when necessary. Your healthcare provider is the best person to evaluate your symptoms, diagnose any underlying conditions, and provide appropriate treatment options to help you find relief from your respiratory issues.

Conclusion

After reading Cough No More, you now have a wealth of natural tools and techniques to manage and relieve coughs. You understand the various types of coughs, their potential causes, and when to seek medical care. You've learned that many natural ingredients, like honey, herbs, essential oils, and foods, can tame coughs safely and effectively.

This book equips you to make lifestyle changes to avoid cough triggers. You can leverage home remedies like steam, fluids, and rest for relief. And you have access to proven natural supplement options that work.

With your newfound knowledge, you can customize a natural cough-fighting plan that fits your needs. Prepare and stock your cough-calming recipes before coughs hit. Know the best over-the-counter options if natural remedies aren't giving enough relief. And advocate for your health with your doctor, using natural therapies alongside or even instead of conventional medications.

Coughs are an inevitable part of life. But now you're empowered to find natural solutions. Trust your body's resilience, support it with natural remedies, and don't be afraid to ask for help. The key is arming yourself with options for soothing coughs of all kinds. With nature on your side, you can rest easy, knowing relief is possible. Breathe freely again—you've got this!